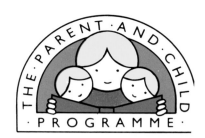

THE·PARENT·AND·CHILD·PROGRAMME·

HELP YOUR BABY
learn

Dorothy Einon

Lecturer in Psychology, University College London

CONTENTS

Photographs by Susanna Price

Helping your baby learn

- Do what comes naturally and you will almost certainly respond to your baby in the right way.

- Watch and understand what your baby is trying to do. You will then see how you can help.

- Remember she is the one who has to learn. Don't do everything for her.

- A happy baby learns best so give lots of cuddles and praise.

- If you respond to her cries she will learn that she can influence the world. If you leave her to cry all the time she may become apathetic, believing that nothing she does can change things.

- The more you share the easier it will be to tune in to your baby's needs.

The development of your baby's mind and senses began before birth and continues alongside her physical development. Because we cannot 'see' that her vision or hearing are no more skilful than her body at birth, we have to remember that she has to learn how to see things as we do and interpret what she hears.

In the same way your baby has to learn how to think and remember. These unseen skills develop just as gradually as those that we can see, and they need just as much help.

Above all else love, encouragement and support are vital. By providing these you give your child the confidence and interest which is vital for all learning. Being in tune with your child's needs helps you know which games and toys will help develop her mind as well as her body.

What should a parent do?

Every parent will respond differently to their child. What all parents know is that they want their baby to be happy and content. What babies seem to know is that finding out is fun. This is why children are extremely curious, and why babies are 'into everything' as soon as they can get about.

Your baby will reach out to a toy instinctively. Around two months she will knock it accidentally, later she will do it deliberately. Doing this makes her happy and excited. It also teaches her about the world and how she can control some of the things that happen in it. She learns that her actions can make things happen. You will know when she has learned this because she will constantly test whether or not it is true. Watching her, you see her pleasure and so set about arranging the world in ways that increase her excitement and pleasure. You tie rattles and pompoms where she can swipe them, and arrange things for her to touch and explore. Later you will probably extend her bath time as she begins to enjoy kicking and splashing. Even without realizing it, you are becoming her teacher. You have helped her to learn the most basic lesson of all: how to learn.

What babies have to learn

A newborn baby does not understand even very simple things about the world. She does not need to at first. As her needs develop so will her abilities. All babies have to learn the same things. They do so in the same order, but not necessarily at the same rate.

She has to learn how to understand what she sees. At first it must be like looking at the pieces of a jigsaw; your baby does not know that together they make a picture. When tiny babies look at pictures of faces they do not mind whether the mouth is next to the eye, or the nose just below the hair. They are quite happy with a jumbled face if it has all the bits. It is only at about six weeks that your baby begins to prefer a proper face to a jumble.

A baby does not even know where she stops and where the rest of the world begins. She has to learn that her own hands belong to her, and that her mother's breast does not!

Playing is learning

Your baby learns gradually, and needs a great deal of practice. Play is the way she practises. The games you play are never a waste of time; they are absolutely essential to your baby's development. Because you know your baby best and can judge what will frighten and what will interest her, you are her best teacher. Until she can control her world she depends upon you to show it to her.

▼Closeness and understanding make a parent the first and best teacher.

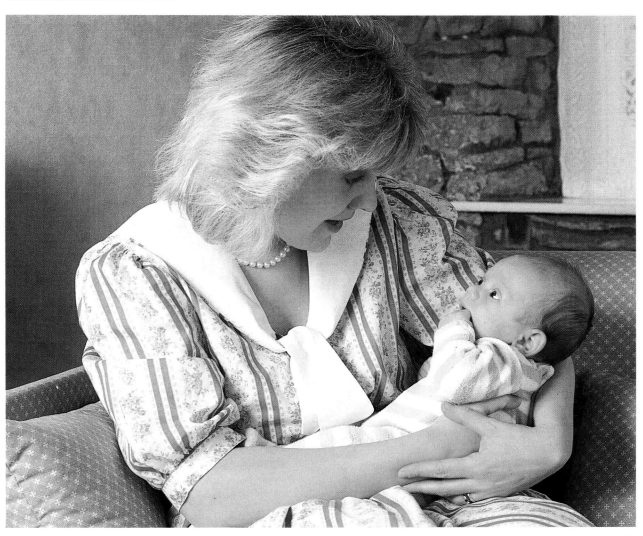

Seeing

● Between 25–30 cm is the best distance for your newborn baby to see you.

● In the first weeks your baby needs movement and sound to be able to find the things you show him.

● From six weeks onwards he will begin to take an interest in stationary objects.

● Depending on his mood he may take longer to respond. Make sure you have (and hold) his attention.

● Let him have a say in whether he plays or not.

Twenty weeks after conception your baby can see. Babies are known to respond to sunlight even from inside the womb. But this 'sight' is very basic and allows your baby to see only light and dark. At birth, he sees best at about 30 centimetres, anything nearer or further than this is out of focus. Even within that clear band of vision his eyes do not see much detail and the limited view his eyes pass to his brain is not made into a picture of the world. He sees only the bits, not the whole.

But if you think about it, perhaps it is best this way. Imagine trying to make sense of the world, all at once. Nature plans it so that the world is gradually revealed to your baby and he can make sense of it a little at a time. He starts with his vision focused at just the right distance to see his mother's face as he feeds. When we talk to a baby we instinctively move close, into this clear band of vision. Even children do this as they talk to a baby.

When he needs to know more about the world, his eyes will focus at other distances and his ability to see detail will improve. At about six to eight weeks he will begin to put the pieces of the world together and see the whole picture. He will be able to watch his hands, to see you from across the room and kick with delight as he passes under trees in his pram. By the time he needs more detail (at six months as he reaches to pick up a rattle, or at nine months when he begins to pick up tiny things) his vision will have developed.

How can I help?

It may seem odd to think of your baby practising how to see, but he does and you can help him to understand the visual world by showing him the things he needs to see. In the early weeks a baby's visual world is concerned with where things are, not what they are. He finds things more easily if they move and make a noise. He will like to watch a mobile and toys that swing and catch the light. Best of all he will like your moving, talking face.

By eight weeks he is able to locate the things he wants to see, and begins to look carefully at detail. Now he is more concerned with what things are and how they fit into his picture of the world. You will see him looking from one part of your face to another and back again, building up a picture of the whole.

Provide your baby with a variety of things to see and reach out towards. Dangle them from strings, fix them to the

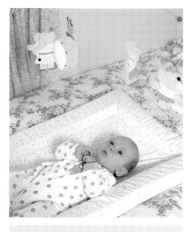

▲Your baby will always want
▼to look at the interesting
things you can show him.

bars of his cot or carry him around and show him things. Make sure that things intended for him, like mobiles, are fixed so that he, not you, gets the best view.

Babies like clear bright colours, simple shapes, bold patterns and clear lines. Best of all they love faces. Make sure you look at him as often as you can – and that he can see you. A mirror (safety plastic kind) fixed to his cot will let him see his own face.

Bright pictures torn from magazines, or board books propped open will be enjoyed by a baby lying on a rug or in his cot. A lieback chair, or carrying him around will give him a much better view of the world once he is able to focus at different distances. Propped up or sitting he will enjoy watching you as you work.

Around three to four months you will find your baby obsessed with objects – handling, mouthing and reaching out for everything within reach.

Although babies need stimulation, they need to progress at their own speed. Do not bombard him with stimulation, changing everything every day. He needs time to discover and explore the things you show him. You can provide him with the opportunity and time to explore things safely.

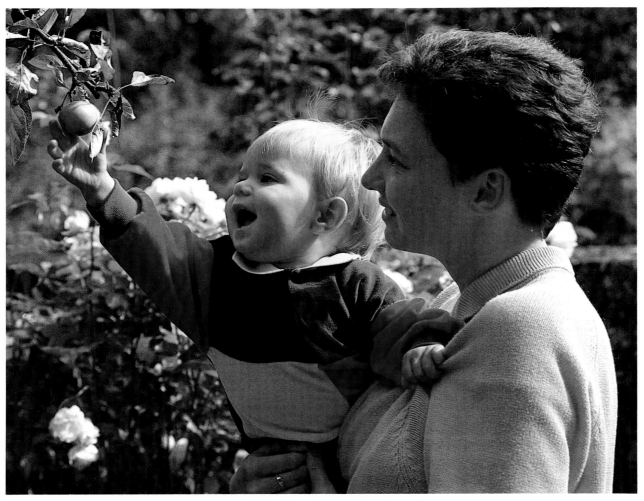

Hearing

▶ As you work, she will enjoy making her own sounds.

Your baby could hear before she was born. She heard her mother's heart beating, her blood flowing, stomach rumbling, her voice and the muffled sound of the world outside. She builds on these early beginnings. She learns that some sounds form a constant background noise (these comfort her) and some, like your voice, come and go (these interest her most). She learns that there are similarities and differences between sounds. In particular, there are sounds which are the 'same' when her mother or father talks to her. Quite soon she is picking out that 'sameness'; these are the sounds of her future language. In three short years she will have learned not only to understand all that you say, but also to say it for herself.

It is natural to assume that babies hear perfectly at birth. After all, they respond to sound, starting at loud noises and looking towards us as we speak. But although the basics are intact, there is still a great deal to be learned, and your child will benefit from a little extra help.

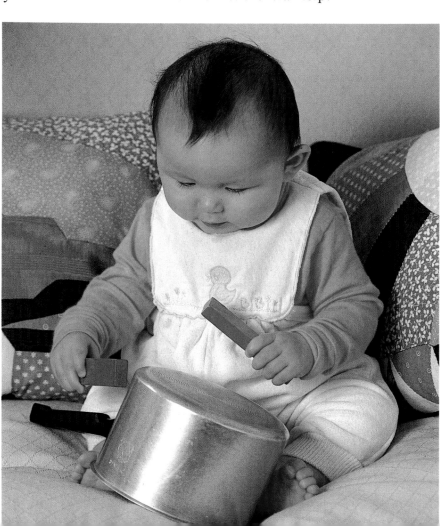

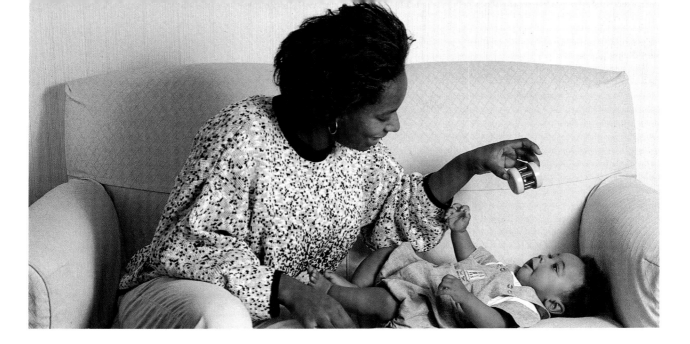

How can I help?

For generations parents have shown rattles to babies, little realizing that they are helping their baby learn to locate sounds. Normally it is hard to practise locating and understanding sounds because sounds disappear, and there is no replay. A parent playing with a baby seems to know it helps to hear the sound again. By holding the rattle in the same place and shaking it again, moving it only after your baby has found it, you are helping her practise listening to and locating a sound.

Sound games to play

You can help her by calling to her from across the room until she 'finds' you, and playing games with rattles, bells or saucepans. Take your time with all these early sound games, she will be quite slow at first. Change the sound from time to time, even babies get bored. Later she will love the challenge of a faster peek-a-boo game, popping up and down on each side of the chair in an unpredictable way. Judge her skill as you play. She likes (and needs) a challenge but will lose interest if you make the game too difficult.

Most of all talk and sing to her, even if it is only to tell her your troubles or sing out of tune. From your voice she learns language as well as how to locate a sound.

Sit a small baby beside you as you work. The sounds of chopping, mixing and banging pans intermingled with your voice give her plenty of sounds to work on.

Because her ears are more mature than her eyes it is easier for your baby to find anything which makes a noise. A rattle attached to her wrist will help her to watch her hand as it moves. When you tie toys to the side of her cot for her to swipe at, make sure that they are noisy ones.

Smell, taste and touch

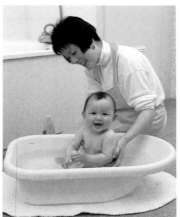

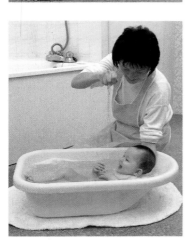

▲Although tiny babies often feel insecure without clothes most love the feel of water by the time they are a few months old. If she enjoys her bath you might like to take her swimming after first vaccinations at around four months.

Knowing your smell

For a newborn baby, the senses of sound and smell are the most important. It is through these senses that she first knows you. A baby can recognize (and will prefer) her own mother's breast pads within a week of birth. If you are anxious or upset she may well sense this through you.

Taste

Your baby probably starts to taste in the womb. She certainly drinks the amniotic fluid. Occasionally babies get hiccups from gulping it down too fast! Since all body fluids are salty it is not surprising that she prefers salty water when first born. But within a week her preference for sweetness has developed. Until weaning, she will only taste milk. After weaning, introduce her gradually to a variety of foods. It is not true that babies prefer bland food. Most are quite happy with garlic and quite strong tastes like blue cheese occasionally introduced into their diet. There are exceptions though, even Mexican babies seem to dislike chillies, although other spicy foods are often enjoyed.

Touch

At eight weeks after conception your baby is sensitive to touch and will move away, for example, if the needle touches her during amniocentesis. At birth she is sensitive to your touch, and she will respond to your kisses and caresses but she cannot explore the world with her own hands.

Feeling with mouth and hands

The two most sensitive areas of the human body are the mouth and hands. We use both of these to explore the world. With our hands we feel and touch as well as manipulate the world. With our mouths we explore the texture of food. Because a newborn baby cannot control her fingers (except to clasp objects tightly into the palm of her hand) she cannot use her hands to explore until she is about nine months old.

Her fingers close in a standard pattern, and she is unable to use them independently. So she cannot prod or poke until about nine months. Nor can she move things about within her hand. All this is needed if she is to explore the shape of things she holds. A very young baby is

● A baby needs to experience different tastes. If you give her totally bland food it will be more difficult to wean her onto your food later.

● If your child finds comfort in a blanket she will probably want it to smell 'right'. Cut the blanket in half and you can wash one half at a time.

● Dresses are much easier to clutch than stretch suits, and they do not get lost when she lets go! Let her wear them in the first couple of months to give her something to explore with her hands.

▼ Until she can control her hands she uses her mouth for exploring.

dependent on you giving her things to feel. She will enjoy feeling different textures. Paper is an interesting texture to give her but **stay with her** – she could choke if she puts too much in her mouth.

Until she can control her hands (stages in the development of hand control are discussed on pages 20–21) she uses her mouth for exploring. It is much more sensitive. Here she can poke and prod with her tongue and manipulate with her lips. It is nine or ten months before her fingers are skilled enough to explore in this way.

This does not mean that her hands are insensitive. They have all the sensation without the skill. She will love to feel different textures in her fingers, and by six months or so she will probably begin to stroke things. Many children find the silky touch of blanket binding very comforting.

Some children continue to put things into their mouths long after they can use their hands. They probably find this comforting. If you panic about this your baby may learn that it is a wonderful way to attract your attention, and may run up with something in her mouth while you are on the telephone or are preparing dinner. If she needs something in her mouth for comfort, a dummy or pacifier may be safer.

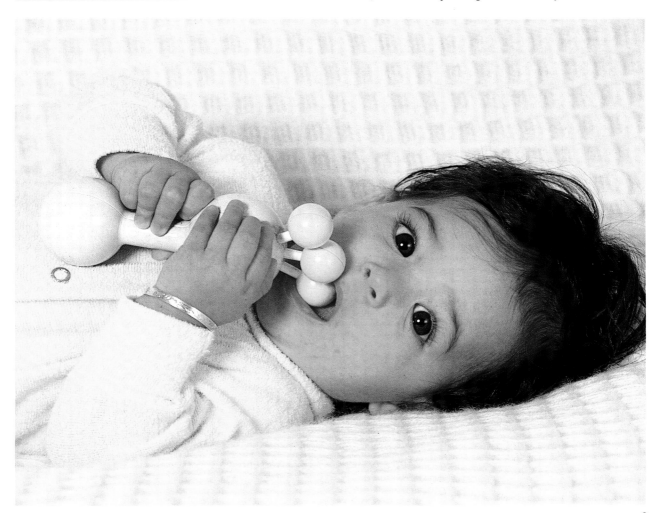

Smiling and crying

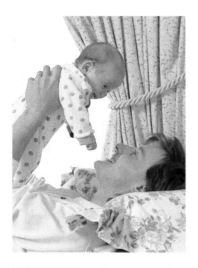

▲ Fun with you helps all development.

Your baby draws you to him when he smiles. Who can walk past a beaming six-month-old without saying hallo? We can think of a smile as a baby's way of saying talk to me and stimulate me.

Adults and children learn best when alert and happy. A laughing, smiling baby is telling you that he is ready to learn. A child who can keep laughing as he learns has a most precious gift: he knows that finding out is fun.

Laughing and learning

All games involving other people and with a surprise in store will make your baby laugh. As he laughs he meets your eye and learns that being with people is fun, and that fun is for sharing.

People who have studied babies have found that it is in these intense, happy, social games that memory develops, and that babies begin to communicate. They are, in short, the most important games of early childhood. Your baby will grow and develop without a single toy, but without these games he will be a sad withdrawn baby, slow to develop, slow to learn and slow to communicate.

Crying

Crying is another form of communication. If smiling says stimulate and talk to me, crying says comfort me and tend to my bodily needs. You will come to recognize his hunger cries, his anger and his pain.

Most small babies cry because they need comfort and are anxious when left alone. Although your child can feel a need to be held, he does not miss any particular person. Until he can remember you, and this does not happen until he is at least six months old, he will not cry for you.

When your baby cries look first to his most basic needs – is he hungry, cold or lonely? Some babies cry from tiredness and are unable to get off to sleep. Being wrapped tightly or lying on a soft sheepskin rug is warm and secure, and feels like being cuddled. Being held, carried or rocked will calm, soothe and reassure and there are many ways of achieving this – from rocking a cradle at the foot of your bed with your toe to taking a short trip round the block! Giving your baby something to suck – breast, bottle or dummy, or something to listen to can also bring an end to crying.

Development of the senses

All babies develop at a different rate. The points below are discussed in further detail in **Seeing** (pages 4–5), **Hearing** (pages 6–7) and **Smell, taste and touch** (pages 8–9).

	Seeing	Hearing	Smell	Taste	Touch
Birth	• Baby sees at 25–30 cm. • Can bring eyes to look at a point. Can follow movement but not very well. • Sees a mouth, a nose or an eye rather than a whole face.	• Responds to sounds; especially pitch and loudness in human voice. • Can tell the difference between some sounds. • Can locate sounds in front. • Will turn roughly in the direction of a sound from either side.	• Reacts strongly to smell.	• Can tell salt from sweet and bitter. • Will prefer sweet by one week.	• Sensitive to touch all over body – hands and mouth especially sensitive. • Will close hand over anything felt in hand. Will curl toes in same way. • Will turn head and open mouth if cheek is touched. Senses hot and cold.
2 Weeks	• Can discriminate between colours. • Sees moving objects more easily than stationary ones.	• Locates sounds more easily than things seen.	• Can recognize mother's smell. • May smell mother's anxiety.	• Will accept a bottle even if breast fed.	
6 Weeks	• Able to focus at any distance but detail is still very poor.		• Likes smells we like. • Turns from foul smells.		• May soon begin to enjoy the 'feel' of water and kicking against cot bumper.
6 Months	• Watches hands. • Sees depth. • Sees detail more clearly but still short-sighted.	• Locates sound easily. • Distinguishes between speech sounds. • Enjoys making sounds by banging and shouting.		• Will develop individual preferences.	• Will not automatically close hand over objects. • Takes things to mouth to explore.
8 Months	• Can look up from what he/she is doing and back. • Can watch things that are dropped.	• May understand a few words. • May respond to name.		• Might have clear likes and dislikes.	• Begins to manipulate objects in hands. Touching and stroking rather than grabbing. • Lets go by opening hand. Passes things hand to hand.
1 Year	• Looks for things that are hidden.	• Responds to simple instructions.			• Will be poking, prodding and pointing by now. Uses hands to explore. • Deliberately lets go.

Before talking

Tuning in to language

Long before your baby can say his first word he is tuning in to language. Within hours of birth he will move gently in time with you as you speak. (We all do this when we talk to each other; the remarkable thing is how soon babies tune in.) Within weeks he will move his mouth as if he is talking, and wait for you to reply. If you talk without pausing or smile without a break he will probably cry. Even babies get bored and fed up with someone who hogs the limelight all the time.

Talking to your baby

You and your baby can talk to each other without any words. With smiles and touches your baby will learn to take turns in a 'conversation' as you respond to each other.

Talking to a baby is the most natural thing in the world. Some people make 'baby noises' and some just talk, asking questions and answering on the baby's behalf. Whatever you do, your baby will love it. You are giving him your full attention, he is responding and loving the sound of your voice. At the same time he is learning how to communicate, at first by smiles, gurgles and kicks and later by sounds which eventually become words.

▼Games are a good way to talk and have fun together.

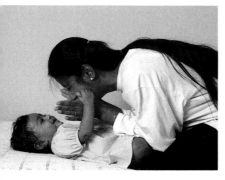

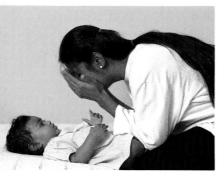

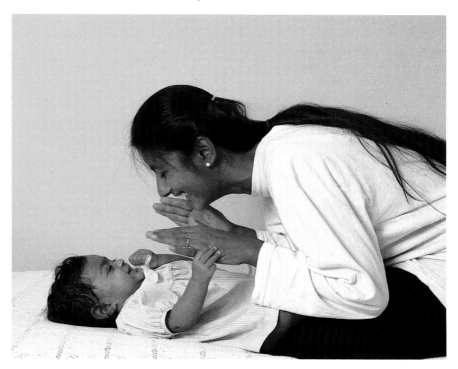

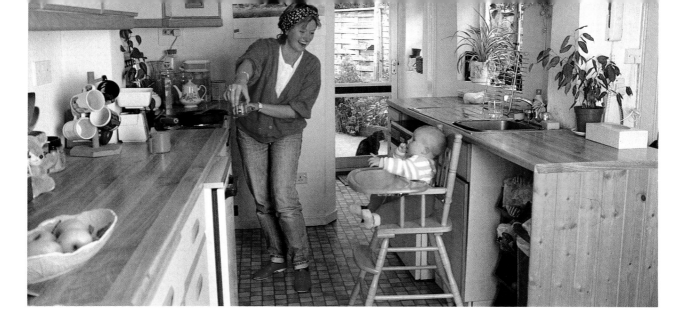

If you are shy you will find that toys are a good vehicle for talking to your baby. Use any reason at all for a chat as he needs you to talk with him – how else can he learn a language?

Moreover, bright colours, noises, and the element of surprise in many baby toys and games attract his attention and help conversation. We have a reason to say, 'Look at this, do you like it?'

Even if you chatter to him all the time you will find objects, books and toys useful. They ensure that you are both attending to the same thing. It is easy to see how important this is to early language learning. He learns what things are called because you name them. You say the word as your baby is 'thinking' about the thing you are showing. Anything that helps you to 'think' about the same thing (like pointing or sharing songs and books) will help him to learn what words mean.

Most parents talk to babies as they shake rattles, play peek-a-boo games or zoom soft toys in to tickle tummies. These simple games practise the skills of sharing attention.

Sharing books together

One of the best ways to be sure that you and your baby are looking at the same thing is, of course, to share a book. It is surprising how even very young babies like to do this. Try it as soon as he can sit comfortably on your lap.

Very small babies like clear patches of colour against a neutral background. The solid shapes of animals (whether realistic or not) are good choices, so are realistic pictures of familiar objects like shoes, socks, cots and spoons.

Name them as you show them to him, pointing to focus his attention. At this stage he will find complex pictures and fussy drawings less interesting as these make it harder for him to make the association between word and object.

TOGETHER

- Make or buy a collage of familiar objects for your baby's bedroom and talk about them each day. A simple bedtime routine can be very reassuring and calming.

- Point out things around your home, show him things that make noises and name things whenever possible.

- Describe what you are doing and seeing together, especially when out of the house. This can be comforting in strange situations.

Talking sounds

'Dada dadadada.' She is looking at her daddy but does she mean what she says? Almost certainly not, she is only babbling. All babies do it. They make the sounds that are used in all languages, but at first they are not influenced by the sounds they hear around them. Japanese babies make just as many 'rr' sounds as English babies though 'rr' is not used in Japanese. Babies all over Europe make the clicks that are used in some African languages, although they never hear anyone making them.

All babies babble

Babbling seems to progress without much influence from the world outside. Your baby may babble more because you talk back to her, but babies everywhere make the same babbling sounds in the same order.

Your baby will start with the sounds formed at the front of her mouth like 'b' and 'p' putting them with the vowel sounds made with an open mouth like 'a' and 'o'. Next she makes sounds formed in the middle of the mouth like 'g' and 'c' and then the ones made at the back of the mouth. She will run through all the vowels in the same way. She doesn't just add new sounds; she has ever changing favourites. One week she will say 'gaga' endlessly, then the 'g' sound will disappear and another sound will replace it.

Making sound patterns

At first her sounds are simple repetitions, then she will begin to mix them and string them together into phrases.

Now what your baby says begins to sound like language because she will start to use patterns of intonation. Raising her voice as if asking a question, and going up and down as we do when we speak. It is the first sign that she is beginning to modify her babbling and to alter her sound production to match what she hears.

Until this stage, no matter how much you say 'daddad', you will not influence what she says. She will babble more, but will not copy what you say.

While she is babbling she is not learning to make the sounds used in language; that seems to come without any practice. She is learning what the noises she makes sound like, learning to match the sound that she makes with the sound she hears herself making. She is finding out what all her 'mouth shapes' sound like.

It is a bit like picking out a tune on a piano. All the notes are there for us, we have only to press the key. But to play a tune by ear we have to know where to put our fingers when we want a certain note. As she babbles she makes every sound that can be used to speak and learns how each one sounds. Later when she needs a 'ba' sound she will know which of her many shapes to choose.

How can I help?

Although you cannot influence what she says at this stage, you can influence how much she practises. Babbling happens when babies are happy and relaxed, and the best stimulus is conversation. A baby likes to babble as if she is talking to you. She will say just what she likes, but she will take her turn, meet your eye and engage in a social game as she does so. Babbling with you will not teach her the words of her language, but it will teach her how to form them, and she will learn that it is fun to talk together.

Songs and rhymes

All children love songs and rhymes. Whether dancing together, bouncing on your knee or relaxing to a little soft music, sounds help her relax, and the combination of sound and movement gives intense pleasure to babies.

Your child learns to associate pleasure and sound, develops social skills, expands her attention span and develops her memory. She also learns the important skill of listening. Children love to experiment with sound, encourage this now and she will carry this love forward into childhood.

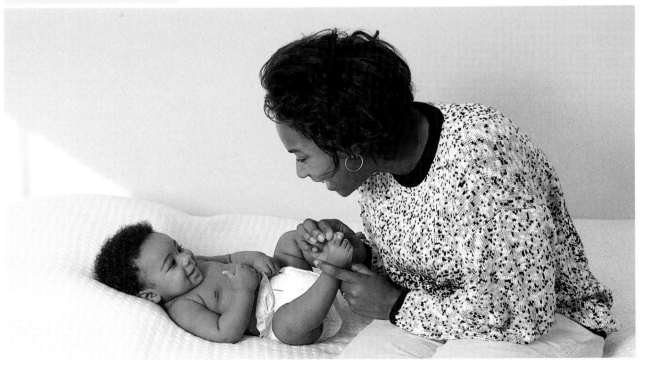

Talking

Many of his earliest words develop from pointing. It is how we direct his attention to things we name for him. 'Look,' we say and point, 'Look, dog! Dog!'

Later he will point for himself. At first he will make a generally excited noise such as 'owow' to attract attention. It will be 'owow' whether it is a tractor, dog or bus.

Words develop next. He begins to use 'tratra' for the tractor and 'owow' for the dogs he sees, maybe using something like 'oo' for anything else he wants to show us. Soon he names cats, asks for his bottle, and points to some of the pictures in his book. Once he knows some names you may find that he wants to skip quickly through the pages he cannot name to get to the ones he can. Encourage him. He has learned that naming is fun and that it is something we like him to do. Don't undermine his pleasure by making him look at every page. Praise every attempt to name something and correct gently by giving the right word when you are reinforcing praise.

▼Sharing picture books is a pleasurable way to learn first words.

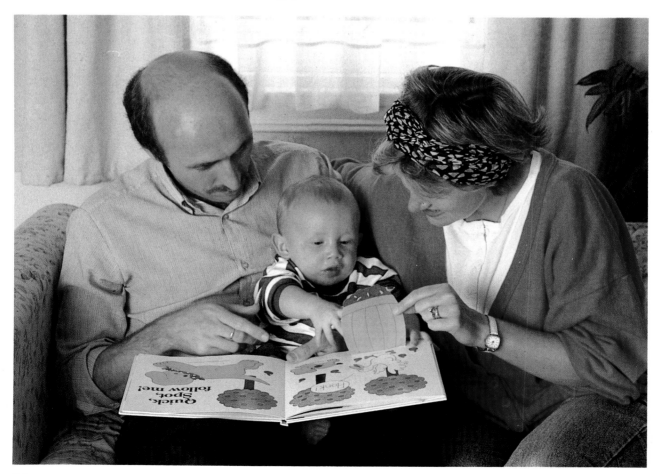

When will my baby speak?

Although the first words may be said at ten months, many babies do not say anything before their first birthday, and some are still not saying much by their second.

If your child is slow to speak do not panic. Unless he has been very slow reaching all developmental milestones, there is unlikely to be a serious problem. Many perfectly normal children find word production difficult. You will probably find that he understands words even though he cannot make the right sounds. Nevertheless it would be wise to have his hearing tested if you have any doubts.

Development of communication skills

Age	Developments
Birth	● Moves in time when you speak. ● Turns to a human voice. ● Prefers high-pitched sounds. ● Prefers human speech to other sounds.
1 Month	● Will learn to take turns in a 'conversation' without words. ● Cries if not allowed a 'turn' in a conversation.
8 Months	● Self-expression through actions. ● Begins to anticipate by squirming or smiling 'knowingly' in familiar games. ● May use some actions as if they are words. ● Deaf babies can begin to learn sign language.
10 Months	● May turn to you and 'ask' you to pick up toys. ● May point at pictures in a book or familiar objects. ● May use noises like 'uhuh' to attract attention to certain needs. ● May indicate 'more', 'pick me up', 'get me out' by actions.
1 Year	● May have one or two words.

Physical development

A newborn baby cannot control her body. She cannot lift her head. The things she can do are reflex actions. She does them automatically, not as a thought-out response.

At birth the hand is unskilled; your baby cannot twist or turn her wrist or move her fingers independently. To do so she must learn to control the muscles of her hand at will, and this takes a great deal of practice.

Getting control

In the first year the body comes gradually under control. The control moves down from your baby's head to her bottom, and out from the body so she controls her arms, then hands and lastly her fingers. You will see this in the way her manual skills develop. First she swipes with her arms, then she grabs with her hand and lastly manipulates with her fingers. The things she needs to play with at each stage in this process must be matched to the task in hand (see below and pages 31–2).

How can I help?

First six weeks The first stage in co-ordinating the hand with the eye is to encourage your baby to look. The best thing to look at is a parent. But most parents are not on hand every minute of the day so string things that she can hear and see across the cot. Select bright noisy objects, which move and catch the light. Change them around from time to time.

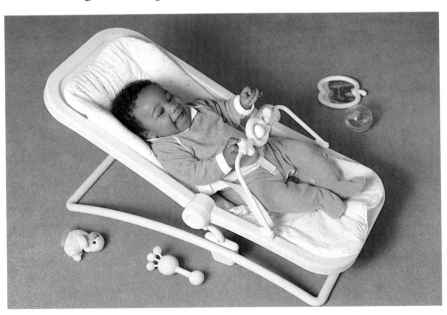

▶Bright, moving and noisy objects encourage your baby to reach out and swipe.

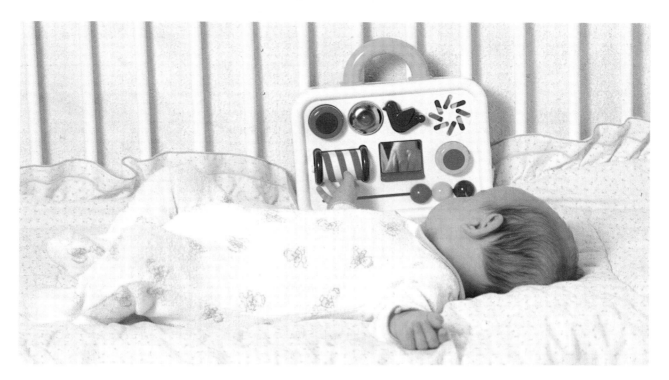

▲ An activity centre provides a wide range of practice and fun in the first year.

A toy tied to the side of the cot will encourage her to reach to the side. She finds reaching to the side much more difficult than reaching in front.

In order to find an object with her hand she must first learn to find it with her eye. (When and what she can see is discussed on pages 4–5.)

Six-twelve weeks Once she has learned to look, she will want to reach out and touch. An object which moves as she swipes at it will attract her attention. She still finds it easier to see it if it moves and makes a noise.

Twelve weeks A baby who always lies on her tummy will not find her hands as easily as one who lies on her back. All babies find it easier if something noisy is placed in their hands. It is possible to buy wrist rattles which a baby wears like a bracelet.

From twelve weeks Once she has found her hands (which happens between eight and twelve weeks), and has learned to swipe at objects, she will be ready to begin grabbing. For this she needs toys to be firmly fixed so that her clumsy hands do not knock them out of reach.

Encourage her by holding things out for her to take from you. Remember she finds it easiest to reach directly in front. Take a brightly coloured rattle with a narrow handle (a dumb-bell shape is perhaps the best) and shake it for her. When she reaches give her plenty of time. She is slow, but let her achieve. Of course, you should help if she is frustrated or losing interest. You know your baby and if you are in tune you will know best how to judge her willingness to keep on trying.

TOGETHER

● Once she has started grabbing, give her toys which are firmly fixed, which do not move away from her.

● Help her to reach out and grab by shaking brightly-coloured objects, such as a rattle, in front of her.

Hand development

Grabbing At first he reaches best if he does not see his hand. It seems to distract him. Later you will see him looking back and forth between the hand and the rattle. With practice he will learn to move his hand to the object. Later he will grab in one smooth movement.

Once he is able to pick things up he will start to take them to his mouth to explore.

Stroking By six or seven months his hand is more controlled and he will begin to stroke as well as grab. Offer silky material, fake fur, and different sorts of textures. Be very careful with pets until you are very sure of the pet and the baby.

Hand to hand At about six to eleven months he will begin to pass from hand to hand, using one hand to work with and one to store.

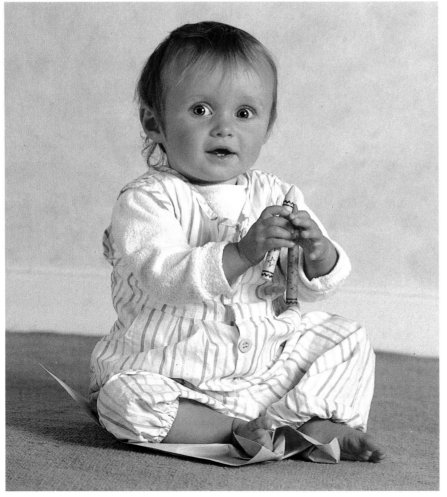

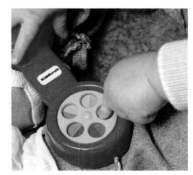

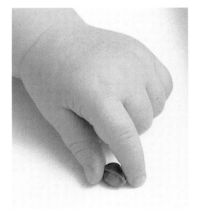

▲Safe toys and food will
◄develop passing from hand to hand, gripping, poking and prodding.

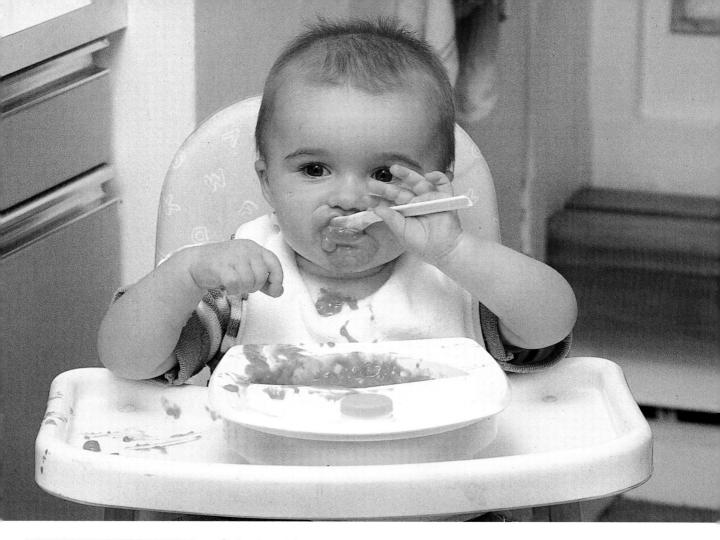

Gripping Slowly his hands are becoming skilled and he can start using them to manipulate and explore. From about six months he begins to use the thumb in opposition to the fingers. It is a gradual process. You may not realize it is happening until you notice when he is opposing finger and thumb in a pincer grip as he picks up a pea. It is safest to use food to practise this pincer movement, try peas, slices of banana, or small sandwiches.

Poking As the thumb moves into position, the rest of the fingers also become more independent, and he will start to poke and prod. A toy telephone, an activity centre or a soft toy to prod, poke and stroke are excellent now.

Letting go In the last months of the first year he develops one further skill; he learns to let go, a skill he practises by dropping everything to hand. He is learning to let go and to watch as things fall. It is one of the basic skills his hands must perform and he learns it, like all physical skills, by constant practice. It is very tedious if you are the one who has to pick everything up. Try sitting him at a low table, or attaching toys to elastic so that he can pull them back into his cot, or putting a box on the floor to catch the bits from the high chair.

Moving about

- At birth her head will flop forward.
- Within a few weeks she will hold up her head for a short period.
- At four months she will sit while you hold her hands.
- At six months she may sit unsteadily without support.
- At seven months she will sit firmly, bracing herself with her hands.
- At eight months she may sit with a straight back.
- At nine months she may be able to reach for toys as she sits.

Development of crawling

- Your baby might start moving by squirming and rolling.
- Between six and ten months she begins to raise her chest as she squirms.
- Gradually she moves her chest higher until she is using her hands and feet to walk.
- Soon she finds hands and knees are easier and faster.

Or

- At about seven months she may move forward from a sitting position on to all fours.
- She will gradually 'step out' from this position.

Each week, watch your baby as she lies on her tummy. You will see how she gradually takes control of her body starting at the top and working down. In the first weeks she will begin to lift and move her head using her neck muscles. Later she will use the muscles of her trunk to squirm forward and turn from side to side. By four to five months she may well be able to roll over.

If once each week you lie her on her back and pull her gently up by her arms into a sitting position you will be able to detect the gradual development of the trunk muscles. At first when you pull her up her head will loll back and will need your hand to support it. Later as she gains control of her head and body she will tuck her head in as she comes up and will use her arms to balance and support herself as her body leans forward onto her knees.

Advantages of sitting

A sitting baby has more to see. She is also more likely to be alert and wide awake. She can watch you as you move around the room, and is much more part of the family. A sitting baby is, in short, a sociable baby. Lying on her back in her cot she not only sees less (who has interesting ceilings?), but she interacts less. She does not beam and draw you into a conversation nearly as often as a baby sitting beside you. As she grows older she can begin to use her hands as she sits, then looking up as you pass she can break from that activity for a moment before returning to play. These shifts in her attention are signs of developing memory (memory development is discussed on page 27), they may be made easier because you stop to talk or smile.

Getting around

Until a baby can move she depends upon you taking the world to her. Once she can move she will go out and choose the things she wants to explore.

Not all babies crawl, but those that do often start soon after they can roll and sit. There is not one sequence, but many.

Moving is learning

Mobility means she is into everything, she can explore at will. She has an entire household full of things to discover and her knowledge of the world expands rapidly. As she

Development of walking

- At birth your baby has a reflex action which makes her step out if her feet touch the floor, but she soon loses this reflex.

- At about four months she will push down on the floor with her feet.

- At the time she begins to sit with support she will also stand with support.

- Soon after she sits firmly she will start to pull herself up on the furniture.

- By about 11 months she will creep along the furniture.

- Soon after she will stand alone (average age 13 months).

- Most babies walk within a month of standing.

- The average age for walking alone is 14 months. The earliest is about 8–9 months, the latest (unless there are problems) about two years. Early walking is not a sign of intelligence.

▶ Mobility means she has an exciting world to explore and you will need to think ahead of her!

TOGETHER

- The best way to encourage walking is to arrange the furniture to give her a route across the room. As she gains confidence creeping along the furniture you can pull the chairs apart and encourage her to bridge gaps.

- A toddle truck can be useful at this stage. Whether you choose a sturdy truck with bricks or one which later becomes a sit and ride car they give years of enjoyment. She can toddle across the room, sit and explore when she gets there, then pull herself up and toddle back.

moves from room to room, her ability to remember is obviously stretched. Mobility brings not only an expanding world and independence, but stretches her abilities to the full.

How can I help?

Once your baby can move and enjoys exploring she will become very frustrated if she cannot reach the things she wants to explore.

She can see more when upright, but cannot explore from a lieback chair. As soon as she takes things to her mouth she needs a chair with a tray, to be propped up, or to be lying on her tummy to play. For a baby under five months a baby bouncer lets her see the world and exercise. For short periods it is excellent. If your baby crawls a baby walker may be useful but not essential. They can restrict rather than encourage exploration.

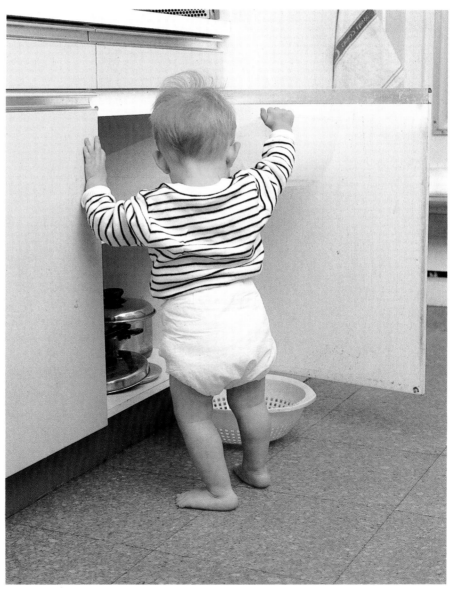

How babies think

In the first two years your baby will learn

- that you are the same person whatever you are doing (object constancy).

- that you still exist even when you're not with him (object permanence).

- that you are one and the same person at all times (object identity).

In the first two months your baby is concerned with where, not what, something is. Not until he is two months old does he begin to concern himself with what things look like. At two months he looks beyond the movement and outline of the objects in his world and concerns himself with the details. He likes the curves, the colours and the parts that make up the whole. He begins to look back and forth from one section to another, taking in the whole object rather than getting fixed on a part as he did in the first weeks. He now sees your face when he looks at you, not just the eye or mouth that he saw in the first weeks.

Things are the same

A baby has to learn that an object is the same even when it looks different, that it has **constancy**. This book is rectangular, but unless you are looking directly at it the picture the eye receives is not a rectangle. But you see and know the book is the same shape however you look at it. You make an adjustment, so it still seems rectangular to you. Do babies make these adjustments? Do they see the breast as the breast whatever the angle? By two or three months they do, but it is not certain that they can before.

Things stay there when he looks away

A baby will learn that objects continue to exist even when he cannot see or feel them any longer, that they have **permanence**. Object permanence takes a very long time to develop. At three months he has the most rudimentary ideas of permanence. If he is playing with your sieve and you take it away, he will not mind, as long as you give him something else. It is as if the sieve does not exist.

At this age it is quite easy to leave a baby all day. He forgets you as soon as you go through the door, you are out of sight, out of mind. The idea that the world exists even when he is not looking develops slowly, starting at about four months and developing over the next year or two.

By nine or ten months, your baby will be experimenting. Many of his games are concerned with dropping and watching objects, moving them from place to place and hiding them inside containers. He will play like this for many months, in many ways, until he is sure that all objects stay exactly the same when he looks away. (These games also reflect a baby's hand development, see pages 20–1.)

Toys to help understanding

● A box or toy in which dolls and figures can be partly or completely hidden.

● A simple shape sorter, or a truck with a lid so that he can hide (and find) toys.

● A jack-in-the-box type toy.

● A bag or bucket to collect things in.

● Books, especially board books because he can turn the pages easily himself.

▶ A shape-sorter will have a long life — at first for hiding games and later for shape recognition.

Things are the same when he looks back

A baby has to learn also that objects keep their unique **identity** from one encounter to the next. Object identity seems to develop at about five months. If you show a baby of four months a reflection of his mother in a mirror he is delighted. If you show him five reflections he is exceedingly happy. One mother is good, five are wonderful. But at around 22–4 weeks infants begin to be extremely upset with multiple mothers, which suggests that there should only be one. It is not certain that babies know that anything else has an identity at this stage, but by about seven or eight months they do.

Learning to think is difficult

Although he has begun to learn, there is still a long way to go. He will play with identity (and much else) in games of fantasy, in stories, in water, sand and toy play. By watching how things change, and in manipulating them in his hands and in his mind, he will reach an adult understanding.

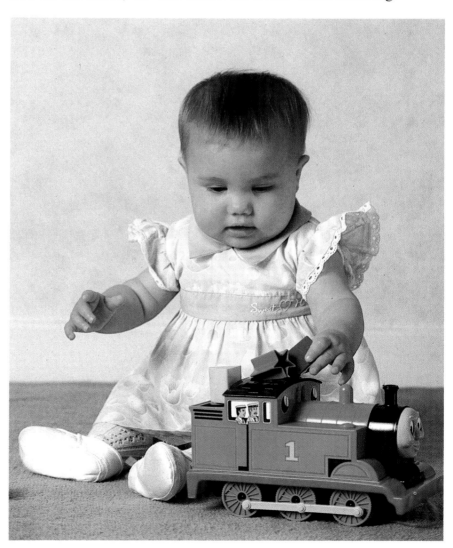

Games to show progress

- Does he look for something when you take it away?

- Does he look if you hide it under a cloth?

- What happens if you let a little bit of the toy peep out from the cloth?

- Does he expect the same toy to be under the cloth? Try making a swop with toys under the cloth. Try taking the toys away altogether. (You will find a stage where he expects something to be there, but is not sure quite what.)

- If you creep around the chair is he waiting for you to pop up on the far side?

- Does he expect you to pop up where you disappeared?

- If you go behind the chair and someone else pops out is he surprised?

Games to help understanding

- Hide and seek games, with toys or with people.

- Peek-a-boo type games with toys and people.

- Looking at books together, especially those with little flaps or holes through which you can peep at the next page.

▶ Books help the development of language and understanding.

How can I help?

If you want to see your child's progress, give him some simple games to play each month. You can record how his play (and thinking) changes. A toy and a tea towel will suffice for most games. Before you hide anything be sure that he knows where it is. Look at the suggestions in the margin for games which will aid understanding and show progress in object recognition.

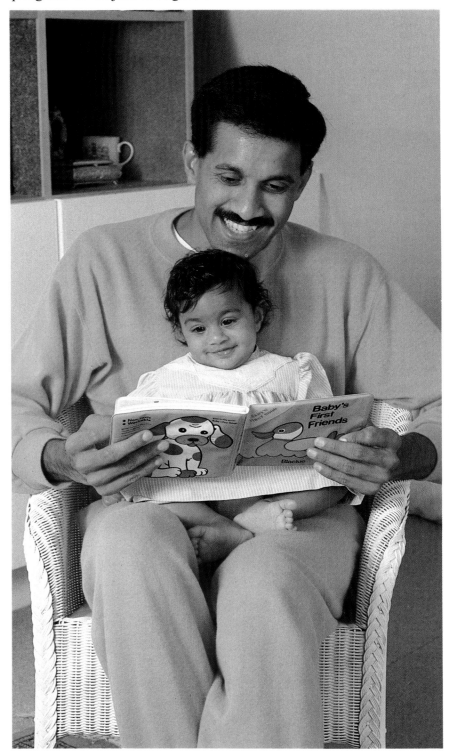

Memory

At first a baby can only learn about things that happen at the same time (like our smell as we hold her). Later she can span a tiny gap (like the time between knocking a toy and seeing it move).

At four months she forgets the rattle as soon as she drops it.

By nine months she can break off playing to watch you and then go back to her game.

More importantly she can now switch her attention between your voice and the things you point out to her. This simple development is the basis on which she builds her early language.

TOGETHER

Don't keep changing her room or the rest of the house around. She needs 'cues' to stay the same. A regular 'guided tour' helps.

Give her plenty of familiar things. The same songs, the same games and the same old toys will help her remember.

Sit in front of a mirror together. Show her herself in the mirror and name things for her.

Anticipation in a regular routine helps build memory.

When feeding, playing and dressing there are lots of games you can play—

— Here comes the spoon (pause) feed.
— Here comes a teddy to tickle your tummy (pause) tickle.
— Here comes a sock looking for a foot (pause) put on the sock.

Most of us know how bacon smells when we smell it, but can't imagine it at other times. All memories are like this at first. A baby cannot 'summon up' anything, even you, until she is about five or six months old. Cuddled up to her mother she smells her milky smell and knows her. But in her cot alone, with no cues, she does not know her parents exist.

Beginning to remember

By three to four months she remembers something more. She looks at the mobile and remembers it can move. By about seven months she can probably remember something that happened in her cot that morning when you put her down for her nap.

The cues of the world around her gradually help her to summon up more detailed memories. You may feel your eight-month-old is trying to ask for a game she played yesterday. By her first birthday you will know she does this.

Holding it in mind

There is another sort of memory: holding something in mind, (like a telephone number as you dial). We call the time we can hold something 'in mind' the attention span. It is very short in a baby and develops slowly over the first years.

Attention span has an important consequence for learning. It is essential to an understanding of 'cause and effect'. If your baby bangs the saucepan lid the noise is immediate. It is easy to learn 'I did that', but not all the things she does have such immediate results. Putting on her coat means we are going out – but it does not mean we are going out at once. To make the association between getting dressed in her coat and going out for a walk means she has to 'hold on' to information for some time. Because your baby's attention span is so short, the things she first associates happen very close together in time. It is only as her attention span develops that she can associate things that she does at one moment with later consequences, like dropping a rattle and seeing it on the floor.

By nine months she will be able to interrupt her play to watch you and return to her game. Once her attention span can bridge a short gap she will be able to attend to an object and to your voice telling her about it. In this way she will begin to learn the names of things and to remember any special interest they hold for her.

Socializing

- Babies do not play together, but they often have a special relationship with other children. If he is an only child he will enjoy watching other children at a parent and baby group, or a visit to the baby clinic.

- Some of the happiest babies make a number of attachments in their first year. He will not love you less because he loves a baby sitter or grandmother.

- Babies cannot understand that by hitting you with a toy they hurt you because they can't put themselves in your shoes. But they can learn that cuddles are appreciated. They can give love.

In the moments after birth your baby will look you directly in the eye, but in the days that follow he may not be as sociable. By six weeks he is beginning to engage with the world, and at three months he is enraptured by you (as you almost certainly are by him). At five months he begins to be more selective with his smiles. His memory improves enough for him to realize that some faces are familiar.

What sociable babies do

Your baby will smile and coo and at three months he will meet your eye and smile and wave his arms and kick when you draw near. His mouth will move as if to talk when you chat with him, and he will start to lift himself as you reach down to pick him up.

Already your baby is learning how to influence his world and your response to his smiles and cries from the very first are teaching him about the world. A child who is treated inconsistently from the start, picked up sometimes and left to cry at other times, has no simple rules about people. He cannot easily work out why he is only occasionally picked up. How could he? There is no obvious rule. Learning about people will be a much more difficult task if some things are not consistent in his emotional world.

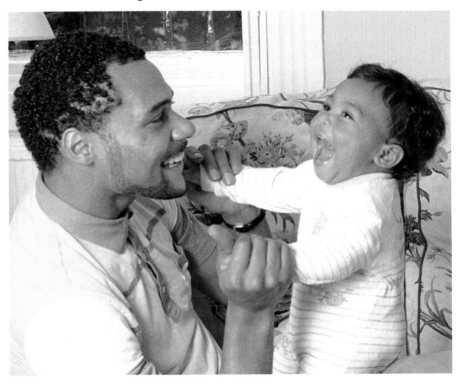

► His self-confidence is built through his special relationship with his parents.

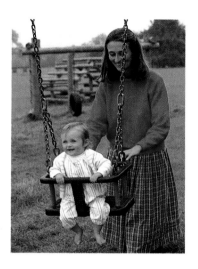

Different babies

Some babies show their love more readily than others, as some people do. If he seems withdrawn do not be tempted to bounce and tickle love out of him. You may frighten him away. Wait. A shy baby needs to be drawn out gently.

It is important to build his confidence, for much of his early learning comes from his relationship with you. It is here that understanding, memory, attention, language and fantasy develop. It is through you that he first learns to say to himself 'so that is how it is'. You also build his confidence and can make him happy and alert, all of which are vital to learning and make it easier.

Getting in tune

At first, the times when you are finely tuned to each other are fleeting, but they grow. By six months he should 'talk' to you for five or ten minutes at a stretch. If he finds this hard, singing, games and play will help this gradual progression. Another small social milestone in these early months is reached when he learns to sustain the conversation in spite of a small distraction. For example, to look up as a car passes and then back to you.

From about eight months you will see your baby is able to answer your questions and make his needs known to you even without words. Many babies develop their own party piece – 'Where's baby's foot?' and out it pops. 'How tall is baby?' and he stretches up his arms. These signs show how much he is understanding and if your baby can make signs he can communicate more directly with you. Even when he begins to use words he will be able to understand far more than he can say.

When he is eating he will be able to let you know exactly what he wants. In the same way when he wants you to pass him something or play a game he'll let you know!

How can I help?

There are many games, songs and rhymes which can be shared without words. Action songs are ideal and your child quickly gets to know when the bump or tickle comes and will anticipate it. Pausing before the tickle gives your child the chance to 'ask' by sign or sound that he wants you to continue.

Songs of all kinds help him to learn. Repetition allows him to anticipate and join in. Often he will make a sign or sound that he knows what is coming and this will be one of his earliest 'words'. Rhyme and rhythm, like repetition, help babies anticipate and join in. Babies can imitate a rhythm by movement or sound.

TOGETHER

- Rhythm and movement bring you together in a pleasurable way.
  — rocking in your arms
  — bouncing on your knee
  — swinging on a swing
  — dancing in your arms

- Rhymes and movement go together, action helps your child gain a sense of rhythm.
  — sing action songs and play out the action or rhythm on your baby's body.
  — make rhymes or repetitive sounds when swinging your child as his whole body is moving rhythmically.

- Music and movement can be used to soothe and reassure your child, or to have an energetic play. The music you enjoy will be just as enjoyable to your child, it doesn't have to be nursery rhymes all the time. Strong rhythms are easiest to dance to.

Finding out about people

It is easy for your baby to see that the toy moves when he hits it and he quickly comes to understand why things happen to objects. His social and emotional world is more complex. Today you may be too busy to pick him up immediately he cries, or too sad to respond fully to his smile. He has to learn that the way people respond to him is influenced by how they feel.

A baby whose cries are responded to quickly is calmer, because his emotional world is consistent and easier to understand. He is able to build a model of people. He begins by thinking they are influenced by what he does. They smile if he smiles, they pick him up if he is unhappy. Once he has learned this he can build in the complexities and begin to understand that when you are looking sad there is little point in expecting a reply. In many ways it is no different from learning that bricks make more noise when he bangs them on the bars of his cot than on his pillow. The signals are more subtle, but they are there.

The importance of social skills

We are social animals, and social skills form the basis of much of our learning. We learn by the experience of others. Almost everything your child learns in school, and much of what he learns at home, will be learned in a social context, in the company of others.

▼It is never too early to be with other children and adults.

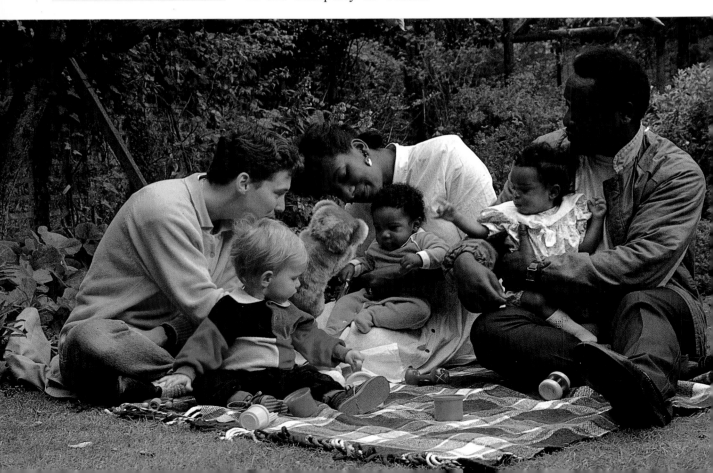

Toys

You are your baby's best toy. You smile, you talk, you move. Everything else is merely a replacement, so give her things like you that move, make sounds, smell, feel and are interesting to see.

Cot and pram toys

faces	● Your baby will particularly like faces, so stick one to her pram or sew one on her mittens in winter.
mobile	● Make or buy a mobile. Some have musical boxes attached. Position it so she gets the best view.
mirror	● A mirror will reflect light and movement and she will enjoy a view of her face. **Make sure it is safe, lightweight and firmly fixed to the cot (special baby mirrors are quite cheap to buy).**
rattle	● Rattles are traditional and important toys. A wrist rattle won't get lost so easily.
teether	● Things to explore with the mouth. Look for different textures and interesting shapes.
pompoms & beads	● Suspend colourful pompoms or cot beads across her cot. Initially, these should move when she swipes them. When she begins to grab make sure they are firmly fixed in place. **Never use long strings, a firm rod fixed across the cot with objects dangling is safer. Always make sure that she cannot get strings or wool around her neck and that beads cannot be swallowed.**
music box	● Music boxes can be very soothing. Some have moving parts for extra interest.
soft ball with bell	● This has a pleasing feel and the bonus of noise. This will be a toy to last for some months.
bright colours	● Your baby will enjoy looking at brightly coloured things like pictures from magazines and board books.
activity centre	● A good one offers a variety of activities which span her development for several months, and teaches her that she can make things happen.

Toys for the first year

books	● Board books can be propped up in a pram or cot. Later, she can sit with you and look at the pictures while you turn the pages. Picture books with simple, clear pictures of animals or familiar objects are best in the first year.
noisy toys and objects	● A drum or saucepans and spoons and toys such as cars or trains which make a noise when moved are particularly good when she is first sitting up.
push-along toys	● Large toys on wheels to be pushed about. When she starts walking a toddle truck will help her.
pull-along toys	● It's fun to have someone with you as you crawl!
stacking toys	● Bricks and beakers have a long life and will be first enjoyed when she can sit up as they won't roll away.
sorting toys	● Shape sorters can be difficult but a simple one can be made with a small ball and shoe box. Cars with passengers are equally enjoyed as she will enjoy putting in and taking out endlessly. An old bag or paper bag filled with objects of different textures is good to explore and feel. **Never use plastic or polythene bags.**
ball	● To play together and to learn to 'let go'.
toy telephone	● At first to manipulate and enjoy the noise, later, as her language develops, she will copy you. A toy with a long life!
surprise toys	● Anticipating the surprise involved in a jack-in-the-box and pop-up dolls will delight her.
soft/cuddly toys	● She may enjoy stroking and cuddling things by six or seven months. **Be careful with pets, make sure they are safe and that she will not grab. If you give her a soft toy to sleep with, as a comfort, make sure there are no loose parts which could be swallowed.**
water play	● Water is enjoyed by most babies after the first months. Lots of fun can be had with floating and inflatable toys. **Never leave your baby alone with water. Remember that your baby loses heat faster than you.**